KETO DIET WEIGHT REDUCTION

DR MOHAMMED MAJEED

Table of Contents

INTRODUCTION

For way too long, we have all blamed fats for weight gain as well as different health problems. The truth is, a diet that's rich in healthy fats enables your body to burn more fats. Yes, fats have been wrongly demonized until now. The ketogenic diet helps change this perspective. It is a simple diet that recommends a low carb intake coupled with a high intake of naturally fatty foods. When you start following this diet, you can improve your overall health while attaining your weight loss objectives.

In this book, you will learn about the keto diet, the benefits it offers, popular myths about consuming fats, and a keto- friendly food list. Once you are armed with all this information, it becomes easier to get started with this brilliant diet. So, are you ready to learn more? If yes, then let us get started immediately. We all have heard of those fad diets like the grapefruit diet or the apple diet. I am here to reveal to you the keto diet that works. A real diet contains a blend of muscle-building protein, energy little amounts of carbs, and strong fats for your heart. For getting in shape, ketosis is the best diet. In a keto diet plan, one would eat loads of protein and fats and little starches to get their body in a condition of ketosis.

When ketosis is built up, medicinal researchers opine the body turns out to be particularly productive in consuming fat and transforming said substances into energy. Additionally, during this procedure, the body is thought to process fat into synthetic concoctions arranged as ketones, which are also said to give noteworthy energy sources.

Chapter One:

ABOUT KETO DIET

The ketogenic diet, also known as the keto diet, is a high-fat and low-carb diet. It promotes the production of ketones by the liver in your body. Whenever you consume any carbs, these carbs are broken down into simple sugars, which are then converted into glucose. Glucose is a molecule that readily converted into energy. However, all glucose is not immediately used, and a portion is stored for later in the form of fats. Since there is no limit on the storage space available for fats, it leads to weight gain. So, if you keep consuming food rich in sugars and starch, your body keeps producing glucose. Therefore, it is not surprising that none of the stored fat is used.

The keto diet helps shift this fundamental process and metabolism. Once you start depriving your body of carbs, the next available source of energy your body will depend on is fats. So, by consuming a diet rich in fats, your body starts burning fats. The shift in metabolism from using glucose to fats is known as ketosis. It is where the ketogenic diet gets its name. The primary idea of the ketogenic diet is to trigger ketosis. There are two ways in which ketosis can be attained- fasting or carb restriction. Once your body starts burning fat to provide energy, this process keeps going on until you consume high levels of carbs or sugars. While following the keto diet, about 70 to 75%

of your daily calorie intake will come from naturally fatty foods, while 20% comes from proteins and the rest from carbs.

Myths and Facts

Fats have been wrongly demonized and often get a bad rap. One of the main reasons for this is the lack of proper information. In this section, let us look at some of the myths and the accompanying facts about the keto diet.

It is a popular misconception that carbohydrates are essential for maintaining good health. Well, carbs are not necessary. It is incorrect to believe that carbs are the only source of energy your body can depend on. Years of evolution have made the human body quite adept at getting used to any changes. Whenever your body is deprived of one source of energy, it quickly looks for alternatives. Since the diet of an average individual is rich in carbs, glucose tends to be the primary source of energy. However, once carbs are eliminated from the diet, the body quickly starts burning fats to provide energy. When you will start Keto diet the primary week 1st week is the principal week on Keto is the most noticeably awful piece of the whole procedure, this is the point at which the feared Keto Flu shows up likewise called the carb influenza.

The Keto Flu is a characteristic response to your body experiences when changing from consuming glucose (sugar) as energy to consuming fat. Numerous individuals who have gone on the Keto Diet say that it feels like pulling back from an addictive substance. This can last anyplace between 3 days to a whole week, it just endured a couple of days for your situation.

While on a ketogenic diet, it is essential to guarantee that one eats inside the limitations of the eating regimen. This is crucial so concerning the person to have the option to stay in a condition of ketosis. Leaving ketosis can be as basic as eating a couple of dinners that are not suggested on the eating regimen. Nonetheless, returning to ketosis is another diverse story altogether. This can frequently take days or weeks relying upon how severe you become when you get back on the eating regimen.

Another myth about the keto diet is that it leads to vitamin deficiencies. Carbs aren't the best source of vitamins. If you want to provide your body with the nutrition it needs, you need to concentrate on eating foods rich in proteins, minerals, vitamins, and healthy fats. While following the keto diet, you will be required to consume plenty of these foods while eliminating unhealthy foods.

You don't have to worry about high levels of cholesterol while following a high-fat diet. All the fat you consume on this diet is quite healthy. Omega-3 fatty acids and other saturated fats included in the keto diet help reduce your levels of bad cholesterol. So, you no longer have to worry about clogging up your arteries.

Another misconception is that ketosis is undesirable. Well, ketosis is a natural state of metabolism, and it occurs when carb consumption is reduced. In this state, your body starts using fats that are stored within. So, you can lose weight without worrying about starvation.

A low-carb diet doesn't lead to muscle loss or damage to your kidneys. Once again, these are myths. Once you start eliminating all processed junk food from your diet and start eating healthy lead, it improves your body's metabolic. When you finally begin feeding your body the kind of nourishment it requires, it improves your overall health.

Apart from this, you don't have to worry about your intake of dietary fibers. All the fiber your body needs is providedfrom different keto-friendly ingredients like vegetables. According to this diet, you are required to consume at least two portions of vegetables daily. When this is combined with all the fatty foods you consume, your appetite will naturally reduce. There is nothing unhealthy about this diet, and as long as you stick to the basic protocols it provides, you can see a positive change in your overall wellbeing.

Chapter Two:

BENEFITS OF THE KETO DIET

There are various benefits of the ketogenic diet, and they are as follows.

Since your primary focus will be on consuming naturally fatty foods and foods rich in fiber and protein, you will feel full for longer. When your tummy is full, the urge to binge on unhealthy snacks also reduces. Therefore, your appetite will reduce. Whenever your appetite reduces, the calories you consume will also decrease. A calorie deficit is one of the preconditions for weight loss. It essentially means that your body is calorie intake must be less than it is calorie expenditure. So, you can start losing weight without depriving yourself of any food.

It helps with fat loss as well. By reducing the carbs, you consume, your body starts burning fat instead of carbs to produce energy. In ketosis, all the excess fat stored within is processed to meet the energy requirements of your body. If you want to lose fat from your abdominal region, then this is the best diet for you.

This diet is excellent for stabilizing and regulating your cholesterol. HDL (high-density lipoproteins) and LDL (low-density lipoproteins) are two forms of cholesterol molecules present within. HDL is often known as good cholesterol and LDL as bad cholesterol. HDL carries all cholesterol molecules towards the liver for their removal. Since this diet helps in the increase of HDL while reducing LDL levels, it improves your heart's health.

Insulin, as well as blood sugar levels, will also be regulated while following this diet. Whenever there is any glucose present in the bloodstream, insulin is produced by the pancreas. Glucose is generated whenever you consume foods rich in carbs. When you don't consume any carbs, no glucose is produced, and this, in turn, reduces the need for insulin as well. Therefore, this diet is a great way to manage diabetes.

It also helps reduce the number of triglycerides present within. The higher the level of triglycerides, the higher is the risk of cardiovascular dysfunctions and diseases. Lowering your carb intake; it helps reduce the level of triglycerides as well.

Common Mistakes to Avoid

Everyone tends to make mistakes while starting a new diet. If you want to reap all the benefits offered by the keto diet, then there are some mistakes you need to avoid. In this section, let us look at some common mistakes you can avoid.

Don't be scared about consuming fats. Remember that your body needs some source of fuel for its optimal functioning. If you restrict your intake of fats as well as carbs, your body will shift into starvation mode. Once your body is in this state, it not only stops burning fats to provide energy but also harms your overall health. Ensure that you eat until your tummy is full. However, the only thing you must keep in mind is to consume the foods discussed in the next section.

Also, be mindful of your protein intake. Consuming excess protein will shift your body out of ketosis. When your body is not in ketosis, you cannot obtain any of the benefits offered by this diet. Excess protein intake enables your body to start burning proteins instead of fats to provide energy. Well, this does defeat the purpose of the ketogenic diet altogether.

Ensure that you consume plenty of water. You need to keep your body hydrated. You need to consume at least eight glasses of water daily. So, make it a point to drink a little water regularly. Whenever you follow a low carb diet like the ghetto diet, it reduces the level of insulin in your body. It, in turn, leads to the excess removal of sodium. Removal of excess sodium encourages your body to start storing water. It, in turn, leads to unnecessary weight gain. So, if you notice that you are suddenly craving for salty food, it is a sign that your body needs more sodium.

You are free to eat everything as long as they don't contain any sugars and are low-carb. Ensure that your daily carb intake is less than 50 grams. If you consume more than this, your body cannot stay in ketosis.

Another common mistake that a lot of beginners make is that they are impatient. Keep in mind that it takes your body a while to shift into ketosis. Give yourself this time before you come to any conclusions about how effective this diet is. It can take anywhere between 7 to 10 days to shift into ketosis.

While shifting into ketosis, you can experience specific symptoms like nausea, constipation, mild headaches, and even tiredness. It is known as the Keto flu, and you might or might not experience these symptoms. Once your body gets used to ketosis, these symptoms will disappear. It is usually caused because of carbohydrate withdrawal. To avoid these side effects, start consuming lots of water, foods rich in sodium, and plenty of dietary fiber. Meals in a keto diet plan contain many essential food types. These are:

Chapter Three:

FOOD LIST

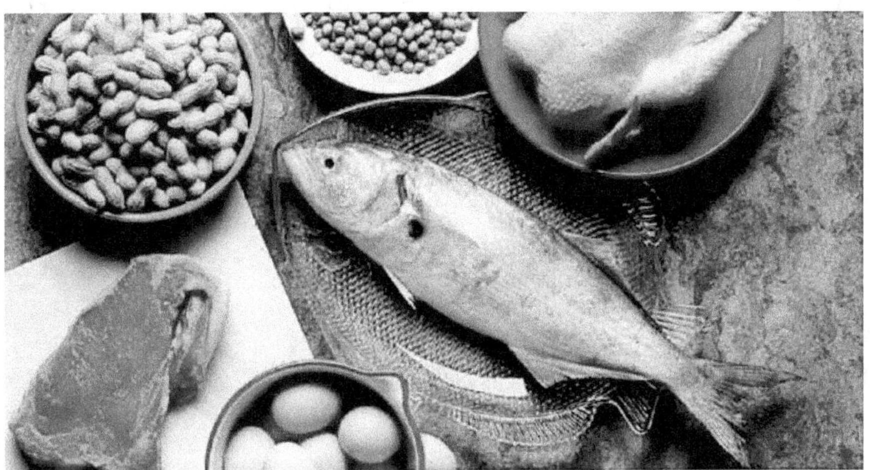

Proteins

When purchasing your protein foods, consistently attempt to pick grass-bolstered, natural and empathetically raised meat and wild-got fish. Aside from offering more supplements, they have not been presented to included hormones, anti- toxins, and other potential poisons.

Meat: The ketogenic diet acknowledges essentially any sort of meat. There is no separation about the kind of cut or preparing. The sources are:

- Beef

- Goat

- Lamb

- Veal

- Venison

Poultry: Any kind of poultry is likewise permitted by the eating regimen. You can improve the substance of the supper by leaving the skin on. However, breading and player ought not to be utilized in the readiness of poultry as they are generally high in sugars. Other than that, you can set up your poultry just as you would prefer. The sources are:

- Chicken

- Duck

- Goose

- Game Hen

- Ostrich

- Partridge

- Quail

- Pheasant

- Squab

- Turkey

Seafood: Another extraordinary wellspring of protein is fish. Fish is an incredible wellspring of omega-3 unsaturated fats.

They additionally have high amounts of minerals and nutrients to help keep you well-fed and solid. The sources are:

- Clams

- Lobster

- Crab

- Mussels

- Prawns

- Oysters

- Scallops

- Snails

- Shrimp

Fish: Fish have great amounts of omega-3 unsaturated fats. You ought to go for fish that are trapped in the wild and sans mercury territories. The sources are:

- Ahi

- Catfish

- Cod

- Halibut

- Flounder

- Herring

- Lobster

- Mahi-mahi

- Mackerel

- Mussel

- Scallops

- Salmon

- Sardines

- Squid

- Snapper

- Swordfish

- Tuna

- Trout

- Walleye

There are different options for protein-rich foods. Whenever possible, opt for grass-fed or organic meats instead of the factory-farmed variants. You can consume fish (catfish, tuna, halibut, mackerel, trout, salmon, snapper, or mahi-mahi), eggs (free-range), meats (beef, lamb, veal, goat, and pork), and poultry (chicken, pheasant, quail, or duck).

Fats

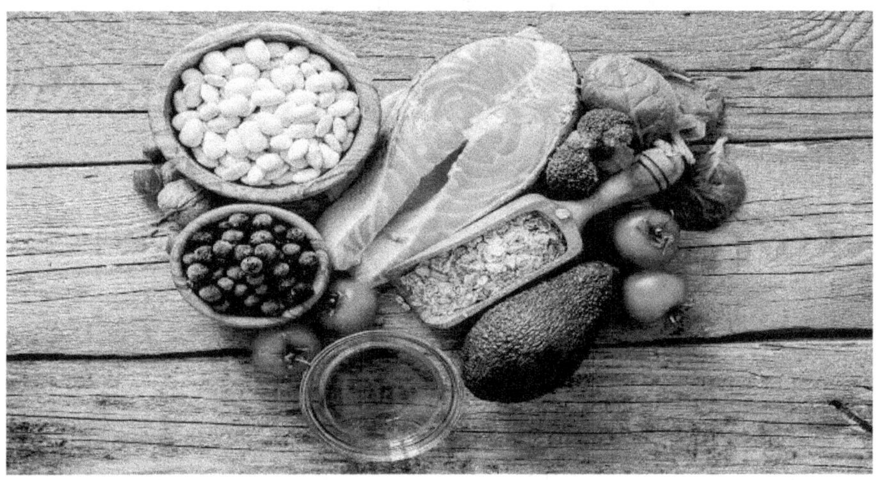

A significant chunk of all the calories you consume will be from healthy fats and oils while following the ghetto diet. All fats are not equal, so you need to be mindful of the facts you consume. Saturated fats, monounsaturated fats, and omega-3 fats are all good for you. The best sources of these fats include avocados, butter, egg yolks, macadamia nuts, and naturally fatty fish. Avoid the docs that contain trans fats and hydrogenated fats. Start using non-hydrogenated oils like coconut oil, ghee, or even olive oil for cooking. Different nuts you can include are pine nuts, almonds, walnuts, macadamia nuts, and Brazil nuts. Ketogenic diets carbs commonly include the utilization of expanded amounts of fats in the eating regimen. They can come in as a major aspect of the cooking procedure or as sauces and dressings. The best sorts of fats are those medium-chain triglycerides (MCTs). These incorporate both MCT oil and coconut oil. Medium-chain triglycerides are effectively used to deliver ketones. Some other similarly great fats for ketosis include:

- Omega-3 & Omega-6 fatty acids

- Salmon

- Trout

- Shellfish

- Tuna

- Monounsaturated & Saturated fats

- Non-hydrogenated oils (when cooking)

- Olive oil

- Butter

- Avocado

- Cheese

- Egg yolks

- Red palm oil

- High oleic

- Beef tallow

- Coconut oil

- Non-hydrogenated lards

- Safflower oils

- Sunflower oils

<u>Some Other Fat Sources:</u>

- Chicken skin

- Coconut butter

- Peanut butter

Vegetables

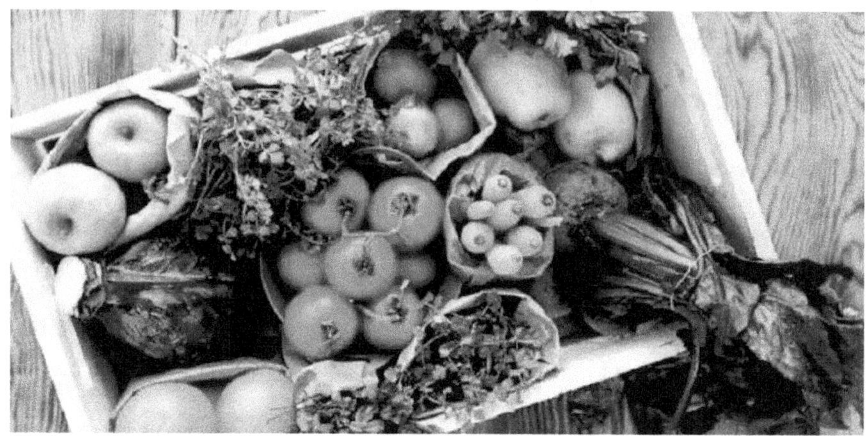

You need to consume plenty of vegetables while following this diet. They are not only rich in vitamins and nutrients but are also a great source of dietary fibers. The different vegetables you can include are asparagus, avocados, kale, spinach, broccoli, beans, carrots, celery, cucumber, cabbage, garlic, mushrooms, bell peppers, lettuce, onions, shallots, potatoes, squash, snow peas, and kale. Stay away from all vegetables, which have a high content of starch like potatoes, sweet potatoes, or any other tubers. Vegetables are the essential wellspring of starch on a ketogenic diet. At the point when you are purchasing vegetables consistently decide on the naturally developed vegetables. Likewise, dim verdant vegetables contain a minimal measure of sugars with great health benefits. The sources are:

- Arugula

- Bok choy

- Asparagus

- Broccoli

- Cauliflower

- Cabbage

- Celery

- Collard Greens

- Garlic Kale

- Kelp

- Lettuce

- Onions

- Mushrooms

- Peppers

- Seaweed

- Radishes

- Spinach

- Watercress

- Swiss Chard

Nuts and seeds

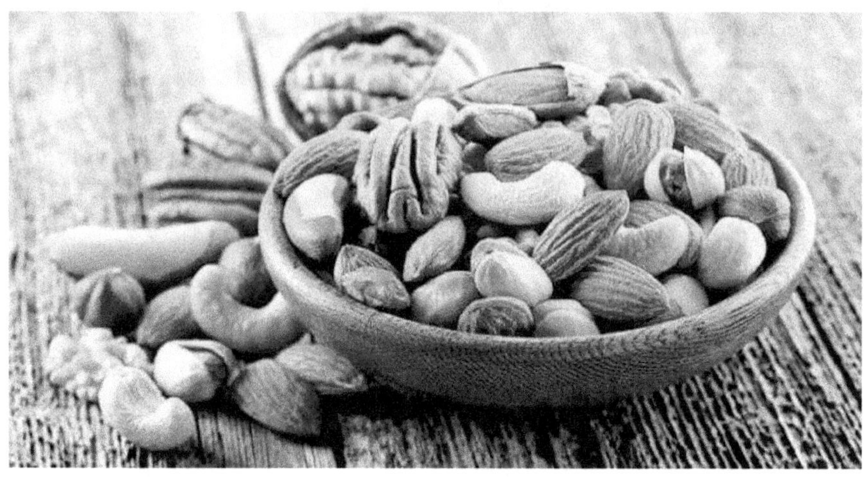

Nuts are healthy as long as you consume them in limited portions. You can eat almonds, walnuts, macadamias, flax seeds, Chia seeds, and sunflower seeds. Nuts like cashews and pistachios contain carbs, so avoid consuming them. A moderate amount of nuts and seeds are permitted on the ketogenic diet. Nuts and seeds are wealthy in protein, fats, and starches. The all-out fat, protein and sugar substance of the nut assortments ought to be checked and added to the all- out day by day calorie computation. Cooked nuts and seeds are the best. Anything that may cause hurt or meddle with ketosis in the body has been expelled from them through the simmering procedure. Nuts ought to be utilized for the most part as a snack. The sources are:

- Almonds

- Hazelnuts

- Brazil Nuts

- Pine Nuts

- Pecans

- Pili Nuts

- Macadamia Nuts

- Pumpkin Seeds

- Sesame Seeds

- Walnuts

- Sunflower Seeds

Dairy Products

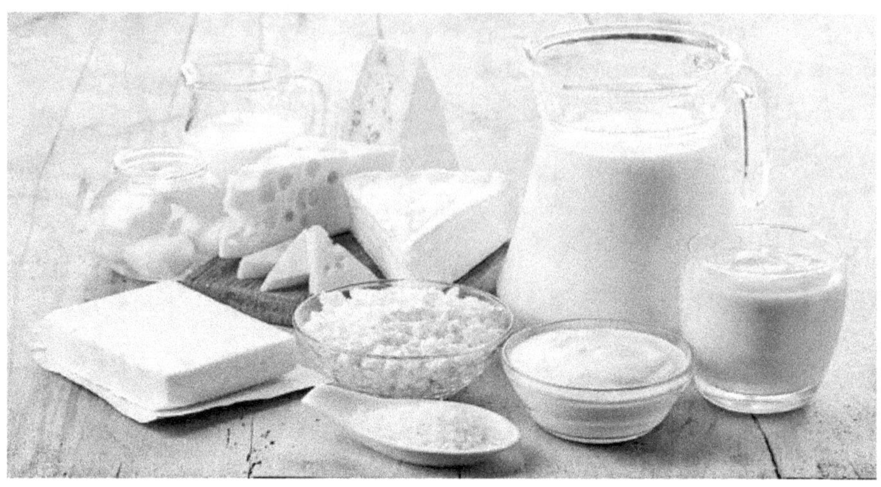

Whenever you opt for any dairy products, choose the full-fat variants instead of the diet ones. Whenever possible, opt for organic dairy products. The different dairy products you can include our full fat whipped cream, soft cheeses, cottage cheese, hard cheeses, full-fat milk, sour cream, Greek yogurt, regular yogurt, and any other dairy products. **Milk and Dairy**

Products

These are extremely fundamental in a ketogenic diet. Grass-nourished and natural sources are progressively ideal. The full-fat assortment is more qualified for the ketogenic diet than them without fat and low-fat verities. The sources are:

- Butter

- Crème Fraiche

- Cheddar

- Heavy Cream

- Sour Cream

- Mozzarella

- Mascarpone Cheese

- Cream Cheese

- Cheeses

- Hard Cheeses

Beverages

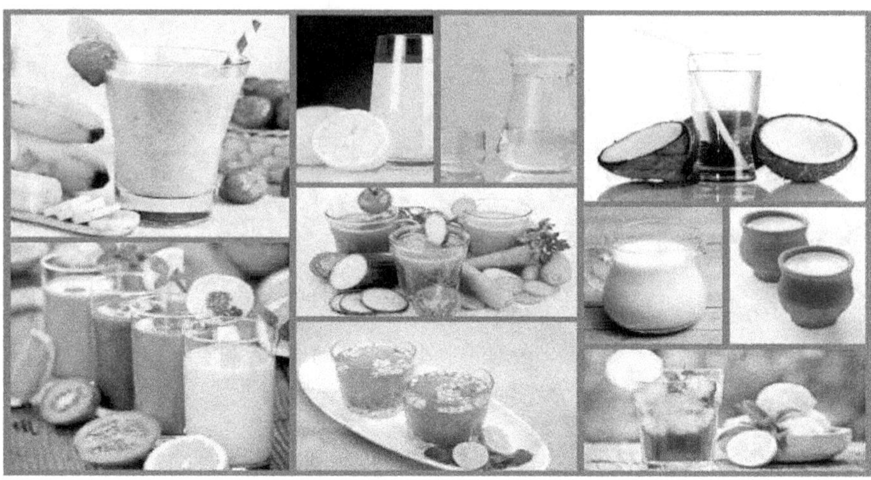

Ensure that your body is thoroughly hydrated. While following this diet. The ghetto diet tends to be diuretic, and if you are not careful, your body can be severely dehydrated. There are certain precautions you need to take to ensure that you are susceptible to urinary tract problems and other issues. Drink at least eight glasses of water or more if required. While drinking fluids, avoid any beverages that contain artificial sweeteners or prepackaged drinks. When you consume coffee and tea in controlled amounts, it is okay. Avoid adding sugar to any of the beverages you drink. Therefore, stay away from sodas, processed fruit juices, and anything else that looks like it was processed in a factory. Instead, you can always opt for black coffee, herbal teas, or even green tea. So Using a low starch diet like the ketogenic diet has a diuretic impact onthe body. Starches attract water to them which causes water maintenance in the body. Notwithstanding, the decreased sugar admission in a ketogenic diet prompts a ton of water misfortune as less water is held in the body and more are discharged. This diuretic impact can without much of a stretch lead to lack of hydration.

In this way, you have to drink a great deal of water - well over the prescribed admission of 8 glasses - when you are on a ketogenic diet. This will assist you in reducing the danger of bladder torment and urinary tract contaminations. Other than water, you can include different kinds of drinks like espresso and teas to help keep you hydrated for the day. Both of these don't fundamentally influence the ketosis state.

The following are some extra drinks you can expend to help keep you hydrated:

- Unsweetened Almond Milk

- Unsweetened Coconut Milk

- Unsweetened Cashew Milk

- Herbal Tea

- Green Tea

- Mineral Water

Herbs, Spices, And Condiments

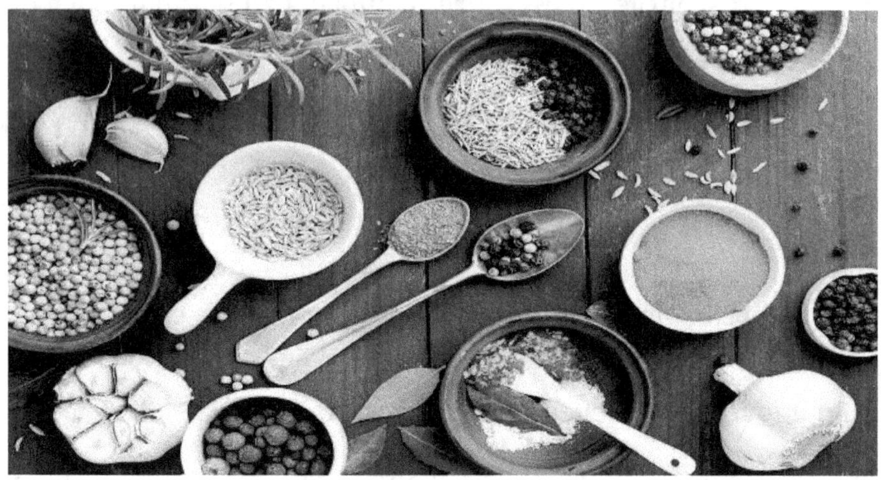

As long as there are no carbs or sugars present, you can consume any condiments. Before you purchase anything, ensure that you carefully read the list of ingredients along with the nutritional facts on the label. Avoid all sweet and condiments like ketchup, barbecue sauce, unhealthy salad dressings, and so on. You can consume all the herbs and spices on this diet.

<u>HOW TO BURN BELLY FAT.</u>

There are 3 things to know –

1- the basics about how to do it. the things that should be added to promote rumen loss and accelerate fat burning.

3- and finally, the procedures that you must remove to lose your unwanted weight in certain places. Losing weight and dieting can be confusing.

<u>Basics</u>

- 3 meals. And if you want fast and easy weight reduction 2 meals and stops bread completely.

- No snacks.

- 250 g of meat per serving.

- Lots of vegetables open and per serving.

- Abandoning sugar. And carb especially bread and honey.date

- Healthy fats (Basic)Things to do.

- Eat daily from your food 70 to 75 present fat from salmon butter fatty meat olive avocado and others

and 20 presents fatty protein meats and Maximus 50 gm 5 presents of carb to get easy and fast shit to ketosis stage . get rid of extra water retention in your body by the use of Himalayan and rock salt and avoid sodium chloride salt and reduce carb and drink too much water and eat parsley and asparagus .drink dandelion tea walk for an half hrs daily least.

This keto plan contra indicated in patients who have liver diseases and kidney diseases and pregnant women and less than 18 years ages

You must eat 3 Meals a day. Maximum is 3 meals a day and minimum are 2 meals a day. 75 persents fatty food

Eating snacks is a not advisable eat, you must get ride snacks. Removing the snacking is very important and vital.

Protein- form 20 presents You must eat above 250 gm , must be quality and veggies to get rid of waste, protein turns into waste product if we have too much of it.

Open amounts of veggies and this will give you the 5 presents of carb give all potassium req. It is going to add 2000-3000mg of potassium.

Things Add to Speed Up with Loss .

Add the following:

- Coconut oil MCTs

- Potassium by eating vegetables or supplement

- Apple cider vinegar: It contains acetic acid; the main ingredient and it is in a pH of 2.5.

Different parts of the body have different pH levels. The key is to know the level of your blood pH and adjust it accordingly.

Acetic acid is very acidic and is used to treat various conditions such as acid reflux (reflux) in which the stomach becomes too alkaline. High levels of cortisol may cause this body condition. Symptoms of calcium or potassium deficiency may also appear, in which case you can use apple cider vinegar.

There are many benefits of apple cider vinegar, and apple cider vinegar is great for all kinds of ailments, but not because of its nutritional content, but from the ability to increase the acidity of the body (unlike what people think) and it will help transport minerals, especially calcium, digest proteins, and stimulate thyroid gland functions. Interestingly, due to the population possesses, apple cider vinegar is a safe and healthy drink.

Metal chromium (a complementary form of food)

B vitamins (food yeast): There are many benefits in taking B vitamins, especially in their natural form.

B1 - Stress and Energy B2 and B3 - Good for Skin, Digestion, Hair and Nails B6 - Essential for the mitochondria to generate energy.

Minerals - potassium, magnesium and calcium 3.

Trace minerals - chromium, selenium and zinc. One of its goals is to help as a cofactor with enzymes. It's also good for hair, nails, skin, muscles, and anything with protein 4.

Amino acids 5. Fiber - can indirectly help reduce insulin or insulin resistance which may also help you in controlling your blood sugar level.

Glutathione - a very powerful antioxidant. It helps prevent oxidative stress in various parts of the body.

Beta glucan - it is very good for the immune system and protects you from viruses and bacteria.

More sleep: Potassium and magnesium are the main minerals for sleep and you can get them from leafy greens, vegetables, and meat. Phosphorous is an accelerator of the nervous system, and it is found in meat and eggs, so too much of it while not eating enough vegetables may lead to sleep problems.

Get rid of bloating gradually in the number of vegetables and reduce nuts * get rid of the problem of food cravings associated with the problems of the monthly cycle of the female

Reduce stress and causes of depression

* Avoid an enhanced flavor mono sodium glutamate MSG / starch modified corn because it causes disorder in the hormone insulin * Avoid food restaurants because of the lack of knowledge of ingredients that often hide their sugar * Avoid excessive exercise because5s9e it causes increased stress

HOW TO START KETO <u>CORRECTLY.</u>

The ketogenic diet puts you in a state called ketosis, which is when your body switches from using sugar as fuel to using ketones as fuel. To do this, you have to reduce the intake of carbohydrates and sugars.

This includes:

- Grains

- Starches

- Sugary drinks

- Bread

- Pasta

- Candy

- Fruits (except for some types of berries).

You also want to limit how often you eat because every time you eat you stimulate insulin. Insulin stops fat burning and leads to fat storage. Our goal is to lower your insulin levels.

The best way to stop the insulin elevation is to reduce the frequency of eating. This doesn't mean you should eat less (or cut calories) once or twice a day. On a healthy keto diet, there is one exception to the no-carb rule. You can eat as many low-carb vegetables as you want

Just avoid starchy vegetables like potatoes, sweet potatoes and corn. You want to eat 7-10 cups of vegetables every day.

After cutting carbohydrates, you should consume a moderate amount of protein. ounces of protein per serving. Meat that contains fat should always be consumed. Never go for fat-free or low-fat options.

You can eat meat, fish, chicken, seafood, eggs (with egg yolks), cheese, and nuts. When consuming protein, you want to focus on consuming healthy fats with it.

Fats will help you feel full and satisfied. Healthy fats include butter, margarine, olive oil, coconut oil, and animal fats.

Avoid soy oil, corn oil, canola oil, and all vegetable oils in general, as they stimulate inflammation in the body. Once you get used to the keto diet, you should add intermittent fasting.

Intermittent fasting is simply cutting back on your meals and allowing your body more time to recover from insulin.

Here are three tips for intermittent fasting:

Eat only when you are hungry

Skip breakfast

Stop snacking to learn practical keto recipes and advice from trained expert

THE BASICS OF A HEALTHY KETO DIET AND FASTING

Go on as long as you can in the morning without eating. Only eat when you are hungry. Continue to fully adapt your body to burn fat instead of sugar. It can take 3 to 5 days or more to go into full a day with a 4-hour eating space - which will give you a 20-hour period to ketosis. Try eating two meals fast and can give you results unless you are experiencing situations such as:

- Menopause

- A slow thyroid condition

- A history of dieting

- Slow metabolism and metabolism in these situations. Cases You only have to eat one meal per day to see significant results.

What do we eat during meals? The first option:

- Eggs (2-4)

- Avocado

- Cheese

- Nut butter - almond butter, peanut butter (sugar free)

The second option:

- Meat (3-6 ounces) 85-170 grams

- Vegetables or salad - olive oil + vinegar

- Nuts

Third option:

- Fish / seafood - salmon and sardines

- Salad

- Bomb / fat balls

The fourth option:

- Chicken (with the skin)

- Asparagus

Olives Important things to remember:

- It is advisable to take vitamins at any time of the day.

- Drink apple / lemon cider vinegar

- Coffee / tea - only once in the morning. Or make coffee with butter (MCT Oil, Butter)

Craving a snack - this means you need more fats and vegetables.

- Craving for bread - you need more B vitamins (electrolytes, B vitamins, salt and nutritional yeast)

- Exercise - the best time during fasting. Adaptation duration - 3 to 5 days or more. The way to recognize you in ketosis is that you are not hungry anymore.

- Fish / seafood - salmon and sardines

- Salad

- Bomb / fat balls

Fourth Option:

- Chicken (with the skin)

- Asparagus plants

Olives Important things to remember:

- It is recommended to take vitamins at any time of the day.

- Take apple cider vinegar / Lemon

- Coffee / tea - only once in the morning. Or make coffee with butter to avoid insulin stimulation . (MCT Oil, Butter)

7 THE EASIEST KETO <u>BREAKFASTS</u>

1. (Greek yogurt with chia seeds) Greek yogurt Strawberry - strawberry - chia seeds. We put diet sugar, we put chia seeds in the water, we cherish it.

2. Eggs with vegetables Ingredients, 2 eggs, 1 tomato, Half an onion, Colored pepper. We cut the pieces, put olive oil, put vegetables, put tomatoes, hot water, choose eggs, and put the cheese.

3. Eggs - avocado Ingredients (eggs - butter - avocado - tomatoes - cheese). We put butter, eggs, Halloumi cheese, chop the avocado Lemon - salt - pepper Iced coffee (Coffee - Cream - Ice Cream)

4. Kaku with microwave oven the ingredients, an egg, 2 tablespoons of coconut or almonds, 1 teaspoon chewing gum, 1/4 teaspoon baking powder, put everything a small spoon of cocoa, butter mix up, 90 seconds in the microwave We put chocolate without sugar.

5. Boiled eggs - mortadella - salad the meal is ready.

6. Bread with iron the ingredients, Eggs, 2 tablespoons almonds or coconut flour, 1 teaspoon chewing gum, 1/4 teaspoon baking powder, splash salt, stevia brush, add here a tablespoon of cheese Its uniqueness is subtle.

7. Muffin eggs with vegetables and cheese the ingredients, 2 eggs, few greens (peppers, tomatoes, onions, and parsley). Add cheese put it in the microwave for two minutes.

CONCLUSION

The ketogenic diet or the keto diet is a high fat and a low-carb diet. Now that you know everything about this diet, it will no longer seem intimidating. It is not just a diet, but a healthier way of life as well. The keto diet will help you shed all those extra pounds while improving the quality of your overall health. Unlike a lot of other fad diets, the keto diet is sustainable in the long run. It helps with weight loss as well as the maintenance of weight loss. All the information you need about this diet was provided within this book. By using a food list given in this book, you'll have a better idea of all the foods you can and cannot eat, to promote weight loss. Add a little bit of exercise to your daily routine, and you can speed up the process of weight loss. Apart from this, you'll start to feel more energized while improving your cardiovascular health.

The keto diet is effective because it increases your consumption of healthy foods without being too restrictive. Now that you are equipped with all this information, all that's left is to get started immediately. It is not difficult to make this transition. With a little patience and conscious effort, you can quickly attain your weight loss objectives. A healthy keto diet plan should comprise about 75% fat, 20% protein, and just 5% or under 50 grams of carbs every day. Concentrate on high- fat, low-carb foods like eggs, meats, dairy and low-carb vegetables, just as without sugar refreshments. Make certain to confine exceptionally handled things and undesirable fats. The reputation of the keto diet plan for weight loss has made it simpler than any time in recent memory to locate a wide cluster of intriguing and solid keto meal thoughts online

Thank you and all the best!